CBD Hemp

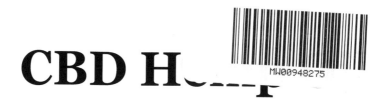

The Essential Guide to Cannabidiol

by Max Burton

Table of Contents

The following eBook is reproduced below with the goal of providing information that is as accurate and reliable as possible. Regardless, purchasing this eBook can be seen as consent to the fact that both the publisher and the author of this book are in no way experts on the topics discussed within and that any recommendations or suggestions that are made herein are for entertainment purposes only. Professionals should be consulted as needed prior to undertaking any of the action endorsed herein.

This declaration is deemed fair and valid by both the American Bar Association and the Committee of Publishers Association and is legally binding throughout the United States.

Furthermore, the transmission, duplication or reproduction of any of the following work including specific information will be considered an illegal act irrespective of if it is done electronically or in print. This extends to creating a secondary or tertiary copy of the work or a recorded copy and is only allowed with express written consent from the Publisher. All additional right reserved.

The information in the following pages is broadly considered to be a truthful and accurate account of facts and as such any inattention, use or misuse of the information in question by the reader will render any resulting actions solely under their purview. There are no scenarios in which the publisher or the original author of this work can be in any fashion deemed liable for any hardship or damages that may befall them after undertaking information described herein.

Additionally, the information in the following pages is intended only for informational purposes and should thus be thought of as universal. As befitting its nature, it is presented without assurance regarding its prolonged validity or interim quality. Trademarks that are mentioned are done without written consent and can in no way be considered an endorsement from the trademark holder.

Introduction

Congratulations on downloading *CBD Hemp Oil: The Essential Guide to Cannabidiol,* and thank you for doing so.

The success began in 2009 when a group of CBD-rich cannabis strains was discovered in Northern California where patients could access medical marijuana legally. The beginnings of the rich oil as a therapeutic option have changed the nation's way of thinking of cannabis.

The following chapters will discuss the little-known 'molecule' and its potential breakthrough as a nutritional component as well as a treatment option for many health issues. Cannabidiol is found all through the stalk, seeds, and flowers of the cannabis plants, including marijuana and hemp.

There are plenty of books on this subject on the market, thanks again for choosing this one! You will discover the neuroprotective and antioxidant properties suggested by the CBD oil products. It is not a question of whether medical marijuana works or not, it is how you can receive its maximum therapeutic benefit.

Every effort was made to ensure it is full of as much useful information as possible; please enjoy!

Chapter 1: Basics of CBD Oil and Cannabidiol

Cannabidiol Hemp Oil or CBD Hemp Oil is stepping up for the debate on marijuana as a medicine. Most individuals already know about tetrahydrocannabinol (THC), the 'high' ingredient in marijuana; but it is now shifting to CBD. These are the two most abundant cannabinoids found naturally in hemp. You will soon understand why and how much evidence is being shown through the medical benefits provided by cannabidiol.

Understand the Terminology for Cannabidiol

Cannabis: The flowering plant includes three distinctive variations:

- Cannabis Sativa
- Cannabis Indica
- Cannabis Ruderalis

Cannabis has been used for centuries for its medicinal, oils, and sturdy fiber purposes. More recently it has been cultivated as a recreational drug since some variations include high concentrations of THC.

Don't be confused; Cannabis oil is not considered CBD oil because purchasing cannabis oil is like purchasing THC oil. It is under strict legal supervision to ensure the sellers don't break the opium legislation. For example, the law could be broken if THC is present in any of the products.

Cannabinoids: This chemical family includes artificial as well as naturally created substances which can vary widely with its effect. Some are classified as illegal, while others are consistent with relaxing and soothing elements.

Cannabidiol is a cannabinoid, but it is not psychoactive.

Cannabinoid Receptors: These are located throughout your body in the peripheral nervous system, central nervous system, and in the brain. With the help of lipids known as endocannabinoids; they form the endocannabinoid system which regulates your mood, pain sensations, memory, and appetite.

CBD: As the second most plentiful product of the cannabis plant, the CBD is a natural occurring cannabinoid. It is still in the shadow of THC because it is safe and legal to consume. Its non-intoxicating components from the cannabis plant have the health professionals, scientists, and medical marijuana patients studying its wide reach concerning its benefits.

Decriminalization: Even though the substance is considered to be illegal; if found in your possession for personal use, you will not be prosecuted.

Endocannabinoid System: This system consists of the cannabinoid receptors and the ones that act on them. It is believed to be another portion of the brain that plays a role, but it hasn't been identified at this time.

Hemp: This is the high-growing varieties of cannabis grown explicitly for the oil, fiber, and seeds. These products are refined into paper, pulp, cloth, resin, wax, fuel, rope, and hemp oil. Ideally, it should only apply to all types of industrial hemp which only contains trace amounts of THC, the psychoactive factor.

Industrial Hemp: The hemp that is grown in today's society—worldwide—is almost all considered industrial hemp when it comes down to the 'fine lines. Marijuana would be considered a non-industrial hemp product—essentially because of all of the cross-breeding that has occurred over the years. Very few explanations exists to fully explain exactly what a hemp plant is in relation to marijuana; in other words. Under these explanations it would mean that industrial hemp is the cannabis plant which is extremely low in THC.

Intoxicating: Substances that cause you to lose control is considered intoxicating. The state of mind can be contributed by any mind altering drug which can cause damage to an organism (the brain); via toxicity, hence the term. Alcohol is a good example for its intoxicating properties.

Psychoactive: The cannabis allows a chemical substance to travel to the brain which directly has an effect on its activity, making it psychoactive. Many of these substances can carry dangerous addiction and side effects when used solely for recreational purposes. The medical applications are also used by physicians as a psychiatric or anesthetic type of drug medication.

THC: This constituent is the most abundant product of the plant and is responsible for the 'high' for marijuana smoking making its production and usage strictly regulated. It is also the abbreviation for Delta-9 tetrahydrocannabinol.

Vape Oil: These oils are also known as concentrates or concentrated cannabis oils. Several different processes are available for extracting the cannabinoids from the cannabis plant. Oils are not made from plant matter but are extracted from the resin glands of the plant. You can also make your own after you have a little experience with the premade version.

Chemistry of the Substance

CBD is one of more than 85 chemical compounds found in cannabinoids found in the cannabis plant. The CBD is the second most abundant ingredient in the cannabis structure, which usually represents up to 40% of the plant's extracts.

The Extraction Process: The cannabis must be dried before you can extract the cannabinoids since you can remove no more 50% of the cannabinoids from fresh material. The material must go through a heating process to convert the THCA into THC, usually an hour, before you can perform a solvent extraction. Chloroform is the most effective solvent for extracting the THC from the cannabis plant. It can remove up to 99% of the cannabinoids within thirty minutes. A second extraction will remove 100% of the THC. However, it is a complicated process.

Natural Sources of the Oil (Cannabis)

As mentioned, cannabidiol can originate in marijuana and hemp variations of cannabis. The biggest variance in the two products availability comes from the way the product is obtained. The CBD established in hemp is legal in the United States, since it has only slight amounts of the THC. However, CBD found in marijuana is federally illegal in the United States except in specific states (mentioned later).

You can purchase CBD hemp oil products in the forms of drops, daily capsules, high concentration extracts, and chewing gum. It is also used in some beauty and skin products from skin creams to shampoos.

Its healthy ingredients include
- Carotene
- Vitamin B
- Vitamin E
- Hemp proteins
- Omega 6 fatty acids
- Omega 3 fatty acids

Where Hemp Oil Originates

Even with the 2014 Farm Bill that passed, you still cannot grow hemp commercially in the United States, even with approved reasons for research needs. Even though hemp crops have been planted in Minnesota, Kentucky, and West Virginia for the first time in over fifty years; the demand for hemp cannot be met domestically. Many of the hemp crops can be cultivated on farms in Europe but must be done with specific cultivars of the plant.

According to the Controlled Substances Act of 1970; you cannot grow industrial hemp in the United States because it is illegal. On the flip side, the sale of hemp products is sold legally in the United States if the following standards are met:

1) It must be lawfully imported to the United States.
2) The hemp cannot originate within the United States.
3) The product material must come from matured seeds and stalks or cake and oil produced from industrial hemp plants.

The production of hemp is regulated and controlled by the United States Drug Enforcement Agency. Therefore, you must have a DEA permit to grow the hemp. Numerous states, such as Colorado and Kentucky, have legalized the farming and research of industrial hemp with consent from the Drug Enforcement Agency. If marijuana is legal in the specific state, CBD can be extracted from either industrial hemp or a CBD-rich strain of cannabis plant.

The interaction of the dissimilar compounds in cannabis work as a team to provide therapeutic effects that aren't achieved by the mixtures separately. Fundamentally, the compounds team together in what is known as the 'entourage effect.'

The Breakdown

You have two plants in the cannabis world categorized as hemp and drug. The essential difference in the CBD-rich and THC-rich plants has to do with the resin content of each of the plants. Low resin is involved with the hemp plant whereas the drug plants grab the high resin counts.

Industrial help varies but is typically sourced from the low-resin varieties from pedigree seeds. The crop usually has a hundred skinny, tall plants for each square meter and is machine-harvested and manufactured into a variety of products.

On the other hand, drug plants maintain the high-resin content with one or two plants in the same per square meter. They are hand-harvested, dried, trimmed, and cured.

In the 1970 Controlled Substances Act was duplicated 'word-for-word' from the 1936 Marijuana Tax Act. The document summarized that certain parts of the plant—particularly the matured stalk and sterilized seed—are exempt from the legal definition of marijuana. The Act did not include the leaves, flowers, and
the sticky resin found throughout the plant.

Resin was mention no less than three times in the 1970 Act. This, making the resin of any part of the marijuana plant, without a mistake, out of bounds by Federal law. The fiber produced from the hemp stalk and oil received a pass, but the resin did not make the cut.

Answering the question of where it comes from can be from the myriad of hemp farmers globally. The CBD oil is a by product or coproduct of industrial hemp which is grown for other purposes. Many of the farmers will sell the biomass to businesses which in turn take the leftovers and extract the CBD. Canada is one of the areas that perform this task.

CBD vs. THC

To fully comprehend the cycle of the CBD oil; you need to understand how the Endocannabinoid system functions. The THC, CBN, and CBD each interlock into the existing receptors which impact appetite, pain modulation, anti-inflammatory effects, and several other immune system responses. There are two essential types of receptors: CB1 and CB2, which serves as well-being.

1) *CB1 Receptors*: These are mostly found in the brain. The receptors play a major role in your motor control, memory processing, and pain regulation. The THC binds to these receptors which create the 'high' effect.

2) *CB2 Receptors*: The CBD binds the immune system receptors to produce an anti-inflammatory effect.

3) *CBN and THCA:* These cannabinoids are lesser known but also play a huge role.

When the CBD is isolated/separated from THC, it removes the illegal and intoxicating high. The CBD is extracted in the oil form and is often located as a mix in hemp oil extracts in varying concentrations.

Both the THC and CBD have many similarities on the molecular level which has led the general public to confusion. Some believe they are the same, but as in recent cases, the differences have become more pronounced. The THC is regulated federally while CBD is regarded safe and legal worldwide.

THC

THC interlocks with the nerve cell receptors but it is different than from the drugs such as heroin or morphine. When the THC interacts with the brain, dopamine is released, and the effects can last up to two hours. However, if ingested, they start within ten to thirty minutes.

One of the worst side effects of THC is paranoia. However, research has shown that the CBD (with 134 users) showed zero results in relation to anxiety or paranoia.

Soporific Effects from THC and CBD: Marijuana is ranked as a superb aid for sleeping manifested in the presence of THC. The bad news is that CBD does not promote sleep, which has been proven through scientific studies.

Key Facts about Cannabidiol

Fact #1: CBD is not Psycho-active: The recreational users do not enjoy the effects of CBD because there is not a 'high' involved with the drug. It still acts on the same pathways, but the THC is the 'high' factor of the equation.

Fact #2: CBD is the Key Ingredient in Cannabis: Cannabis breeders have managed to create a variety that has near zero THC levels and higher levels of CBD. However, rare they are, but popularity has been peaking over the last several years.

Fact #3: The Negative Effects of THC are reduced by CBD: THC causes exhilaration by tying to distinctive CB1 and CB2 nerve receptors in your brain. The CBD doesn't bind these receptors.

Fact #3: CBD from Hemp is Legal: In some states, marijuana grown is legal, but not in all of them. The industrial hemp or medical marijuana plants can be grown and imported legally into the United States. This process makes it much simpler to receive the CBD treatment without breaking the laws. (More on that later.)

Fact #4: Levels Vary with Cannabinoids: Recreational Marijuana plants are grown to be 'high' in THC with varied quantities of CBD, whereas, the industrial hemp plants are lower in THC.

Fact #5: Benefits the Mind: Psychosis can be combatted as well as depression and anxiety disorders.

Fact #6: Has Medical Value: CBD has many values described in detail in Chapter 2 (more on this later).

Fact #7: The Prescription Story: Individuals must have a prescription to order CBD products made from medical marijuana in the state where it is legal to purchase the medical product. You can order CBD from industrial hemp plants online without a prescription.

Fact #8: Easily Accessible and Easy to Use: CBD oil from industrial hemp is legal in most developed countries and all 50 states at the federal level, unlike CBD from cannabis. You will see later how medical marijuana depends on state laws.

You will also discover since some of the hemp oil products do not contain THC, the job-related drug screens will be negated. The CBD hemp oil is extracted with CO_2 extraction methods which keeps the purity of the plant.

How Long CBD Takes to Work

The use of CBD can take anywhere from a few minutes to a few hours to properly get into your system, depending on the dosage, the method used, and the symptoms which you are attempting to combat.

Vaping is the fastest and easiest way to receive the product and can be accomplished with the purchase of a vape starter kit. You can get relief within a few minutes for anxiety as an example.

Applying topically will lead to a more uniform but slower absorption to last for longer periods of time.

If you try hemp oil or chocolate products, it could take twenty minutes to an hour depending on how long it has been since you had your last meal. For faster relief, it is best taken on an empty stomach. If you drink the oil or put it in food, it will take longer for the effects, but you can eliminate the possibilities of dysphoria or headaches.

If you are a first timer, you probably don't know what to expect since there is not a 'high' to trigger the thought pattern. It is only after you realize the ailment is better or you are feeling better about any given situation that you get it.

After a while, you will begin to recognize the subtle calming effect or realize the 'edge' is off of the problem only minutes after administering the oil in whatever form you choose.

Everyone is different, so it may take you longer or less time than anyone else who you might know that is using the medication. You have to experiment with the oils. But remember, start with lower doses, and build up a resistance first. As with any new plan, it is advisable to consult a physician you know and trust, especially if you take other medication or suffer from chronic illnesses.

Chapter 2: Health Benefits of CBD Oil

With all of its benefits, the list could go on forever to praise the many benefits of CBD oil. It is with *HOPE* that we find a way to make this necessary oil available to those who truly need it. This is the basic list of how scientific research has indicated how beneficial the oil is for your body as well as what ailments can be relieved:

Alcohol-Induced Damage: When consumed in large quantities, alcohol exposes your vital organs such as the kidneys and liver to extensive damage. The oil has specific properties which can protect them from this type of excessive abuse. It prevents the fat and lipid accumulation in the liver which can lead to issues including cirrhosis.

Analgesic/Pain Killer: As an analgesic, the CBDs bind to the CB1 receptors to relieve pain throughout your body. Rheumatoid Arthritis is one inflammation in the joints that can be relieved with the use of the CBD Oil. The painful and sometimes immobility issues involving the ankles, fingers, wrists, and feet can receive some relief.

Similar conditions such as osteoarthritis and gout have also received benefits from the hemp oil with the CBD which is removed from the medical marijuana plants. This was scientifically proven to provide a natural treatment in a study in 2006 involving patients with rheumatoid arthritis receiving the oil for five weeks.

Anticonvulsant: Can suppress seizure activity

Antiemetic: CBDs can reduce vomiting and nausea; making this useful during treatments for serious diseases such as individuals who are enduring chemotherapy. It is also useful if you suffer from motion sickness, certain smells, or even the weather. This could be the cure you are seeking if you don't have any apparent reason for the queasiness.

Anti-inflammatory: The oil can combat inflammation disorders which can result in the reduction of swelling.

Anti-oxidant: The oil can combat neurodegenerative disorders and exceeds Vitamin E and Vitamin C in its intensity. When your tissues use oxygen to burn the food you consume as fuel, the result produces unstable particles which have negative effects on your tissues. The CBD oil will give the protection to fight against the stress and inflammation that these radicals induce.

Anti-cancer/Anti-tumor: CBD oil can combat cancer and tumor cells according to several studies using rats and mice for the chosen test candidate. The drug can induce the tumor cell death, inhibit cancer cell growth, and control or inhibit the spread of the cancer cells.

Anti-depressant/Anxiolytic: The oil can alleviate severe social anxiety disorders including depression PTSD, SAD or Generalized Social Anxiety Disorder, and other anxiety disorders that can impair your excellence of life. Unlike pharmaceutical drugs, CBD oil is not addictive and won't harm your kidneys or liver even if it is used for an extended amount of time.

Some marijuana users criticize about an amplified anxiety when smoking. This can be caused by the lowered levels of the CBD in relation to the higher levels of THC found in the marijuana.

Diabetes: If you suffer from diabetes, you will discover cannabinoids are effective in treating the chronic pain revolving around eye disorders, sleep disorders, and other ailments the disease creates on a daily basis.

Digestive Aid: To have a healthy body, you have to have a healthy appetite, especially when your body is attempting to heal itself from illness. According to the National Cancer Institute, CBD oil will stimulate your appetite since your body binds the CBDs to cannabinoid receptors in your body. The CBDs will stimulate your appetite when they 'dock' onto the receptors.

Energy Booster: In the event you feel tired all of the time, it is best to visit your doctor to see if there are any underlying physical ailments that could be causing the lack of energy. On the flip side, you may just need a booster, whereas CBD oil can promote the wakefulness for your body throughout the day. It strengthens your body's cells to ensure they are working correctly and in good shape all of the time.

Epilepsy Treatment: It is unfortunate that many states have implemented medical cannabis programs that prevented patients from receiving the needed cannabis treatments. Until the programs are updated, patients will continue to suffer from these types of ailments from the dreaded disease:

- Absence will create lapses in the person's consciousness.
- Myoclonic creates lurching (isolated) or sporadic movements.
- Clonic symptoms are continued twitching movements.
- Tonic symptoms involve rigidity and muscle stiffness.
- Atonic will cause the least severe type of seizure which involves the loss of muscle tone.
- Grand Mall is characterized by unconsciousness, full-body convulsions, and muscle rigidity. This is the most debilitating and severe category of epilepsy.

The only alternatives are medications carry side effects and are generally ineffective. Some of the pharmaceutical drugs include Depakote, Klonopin, Mysoline, Dilantin, or Tegretol. These would be a thing of the past with the CDB oil which would be one of the most effective and powerful medicines possible to remedy a wide variety of these seizure disorders; all of this over a 'minor semantic' discrepancy.

Cardiovascular diseases can be prevented with the boost daily of 15 to 20 grams of hemp seed or hemp seed oil.

Multiple Sclerosis (MS): If you have a prescription for cannabidiol; you can acquire a mouth spray that contains a proportion of 1:1 with CBD and THC. The mouth spray benefits in these ways: reduction in muscle spasms, reduction in neuropathic pain, reduction in spasticity, and a reduction in sleep disturbances.

The drug is available in at least 15 different countries for the treatment of MS. These are some of the strains that would benefit you including Harlequin, Charlotte's Web, AC/DC, Cannatonic, and Sour Tsunami. You can also consider other products that maintain a high CBD Concentration/Ratio. Out of the current list, it seems Cannatonic seems to be the best option for patients suffering from MS.

These are some tips for taking CBD if you have MS:

- Take your pill during the daytime hours to help keep the symptoms under control without placing yourself at the risk of being 'high' either.
- You can relieve the pain if you vaporize high CBD cannabis, but be sure not to operate a vehicle directly after the consumption.
- Consume a CBD-rich edible product before you retire for the evening for sleep. You might not be able to function properly if you take it during the daylight hours.
- Purchasing the cannabis juice is recommended if you can purchase it in your area.

Schizophrenia and Psychosis: As a psychiatric term, an abnormal state of mind means you have lost contact with reality, meaning you are suffering from psychosis. It is not only a symptom of the schizophrenia and other mood disorders. No risk is involved according to recent studies since it does not contain the concentrated or pure THC.

A common drug that is used for schizophrenia and psychosis is known as amisulpride which has side effects such as enhanced levels of prolactin and weight gain, not evident with CBD oil. As a reoccurring factor that needs to be mentioned; Dopamine 2 over-activity is a main cause associated with mental conditions such as these.

Studies have shown Anandamide, an endogenous cannabinoid, counteracts the over-activity. The oil increases this activity.

Beneficial for Your Skin and Hair: The fatty acids in hemp oil are beneficial for your skin if used in the right proportions. Hemp oil is the main ingredient in many body creams and face creams. You can also benefit from hair oils, conditioners, and shampoos using hemp oil. You can also reduce the loss of hair.

Spinal Injuries: It has been known to lessen tremors. (More benefits in proven research.)

Weight Management: You are concerned with two elements if you decide to lose some weight: physical exercise and food intake. The oil is an excellent metabolism stabilizer which becomes crucial when it comes to physical exercise.

You will also benefit from the suppressed craving for food. If your eating issues are from stress and anxiety, the oil will help eliminate those feelings so you can begin a better eating pattern.

Proven Research

Acne: A study with the *National Institute of Health* published in the *Journal of Clinical Investigation* discovered CBD used on the human sebaceous glands reduced the issues of acne as an anti-inflammatory agent. The oil can inhibit the production of sebum or sebocytes.

SAD Case Study in 2011: A study of 24 individuals was performed who suffered from SAD, and had not tried to seek treatment. The study participants were separated into two groups. One group received a placebo, and the other received 600 mg of CBD. The test was given as an exercise of delivering a speech test. The heart rate, blood pressure, and measurements of psychological and physiological stress were measured.

In comparison, the placebo group presented with more cognitive discomfort and impairment with higher anxiety levels. The CBD may work better than other antidepressants because they have no side effects, acts quickly, and the patient/individual does not suffer from any withdrawal symptoms.

Breast Cancer: According to another study provided by the California Pacific Medical Center, the oil can literally 'turn off' the gene that spreads breast cancer. The ID-1 prevents the cells from reaching to your tissues.

Cardiovascular Disease: According to animal trials, if CBD is administered within a few minutes of a heart attack, it was found to greatly reduce the cell death, inflammation, oxidative stress, and fibrosis as well as preserve the left ventricle's performance. It is also capable of restoring a regular rhythm following a warning stroke or mini-stroke otherwise called an ischemic attack.

You can receive an improved biochemical, neuro behavior, as well as a functional recovery if CBD is administered shortly after a stroke because it protects astrocytes and neurons from damage.

Cigarette Addiction: Twenty-four participants were involved in a double-blind placebo-controlled study. The result was a 40% reduction of the desire to have a cigarette after the use of the inhaler, reducing the desire for nicotine. Therefore, the withdrawal process was made much simpler.

Fibromyalgia: A study using 56 participants were involved in a 2011 study using traditional methods for pain management and others used the CBD. The results of the CBD were observed as greatly improved.

Heart and Blood Pressure Conditions: Rodriguez-Leyva & Pierce discovered the benefits of omega-3 and omega-6 which can decrease heart disease since it contains less that .3% of THC; there won't be any psychoactive properties. It was discovered to have zinc, iron, calcium sulfur, magnesium, sodium, phosphorus, and potassium.

Arginine is in CBD oil making the amino acid do its job of keeping the blood pressure in line. The oils are similar to the nutrients in flaxseed and salmon. It was discovered to reduce atherosclerosis, coronary heart disease, and high blood pressure.

Schizophrenia Treatment: Research provided in Germany by the University of Cologne has also indicated CBD as a benefit to relieve psychotic symptoms relating to schizophrenia. It is estimated that 2.4 million adults suffer from this disease which is about 1.2% of the population.

Children with Seizures: Permission has been granted by the U.S. Food and Drug Administration (FDA) to the University of California in San Francisco for a study of the effect of the use of the purified cannabidiol drug. The applicants are between one and eighteen years of age; all suffering symptoms that are resistant to the methods tried on a conventional scale.

Early childhood conditions, such as the Dravet Syndrome was included with some of the participants during the study. The FDA is closely monitoring this research. Upon approval, more institutions will surely take the lead and provide more studies for the cause.

Negative Effects of THC: The *British Journal of Psychiatry* indicated through research the CBD prevents the THC memory impairments. It helps ease the negative side effects such as paranoia induced by the THC.

Parkinson's disease: A team of researchers from Brazil proved that daily cannabidiol treatments improved the quality of life and well-being. The study covered six weeks where 21 patients received CBD in gelatin capsules. Their doses were given with a placebo, 75 mg daily, and 300 mg per day. The testing proved the treatments helped the symptoms.

Spinal Cord Injuries and CBD Oil: Twelve volunteers provided a 2010 study at the University of Manitoba, Canada to alleviate their spasticity using Nabilone, a synthetic cannabinoid. The Department of Medicine showed eleven out of the twelve patients showed a huge decrease in their affected muscle groups.

The Epidiolex Study

The FDA is also undergoing an 'orphan drug' study for the treatment of pediatric epilepsy called Epidiolex, derived from pure CBD extract. GW Pharmaceuticals is committed to discovering treatment options to treat treatment-resistant or rare conditions for epilepsy conditions. The conditions considered include Lennox-Gastaut Syndrome (LGS), Dravet Syndrome, Infantile Spasms (IS), and Tuberous Sclerosis Complex (TSC).

The series of clinical trials will provide the FDA and other regulatory authorities worldwide with efficacy and safety data which is essential to be considered for an approval of any prescription medication. Some patients will receive a placebo or Epidiolex in addition to his/her current treatment. The plan will be 'blind' studies whereas the patients, physicians, or families will not know which treatment has been assigned to them.

There are currently three phases of trials; one is for IS, one for TSC, and two in LGS. There have been significant reductions for patients, one for the LGS and one for the Dravet Syndrome.

If you are interested in more information, check with <u>this link</u> to see if you qualify.

Infantile spasms or IS occurs in young children and is a rare seizure disorder. It can occur from approximately four months or up to two years. Lennox-Gastaur syndrome can cause a broad range of brain dysfunction resulting in behavioral, cognitive, and psychiatric symptoms. Many times the patient, many times a child, has multiple and often difficult seizures to control.

These are some of the issues involved with Dravet Syndrome which is a catastrophic, rare and lifelong disease that could benefit from the CDB oil:

- Frequent and prolonged seizures
- Balance and movement issues
- Nutrition and growth issues
- Chronic infections
- Sleeping difficulties

These patients suffer and face a 15% to 20% mortality rate because of Sudden Unexplained Death in Epilepsy (SUDEP).

As of December 2015, 261 patients who have been receiving Epidiolex show promising signals as to progress in reducing seizure activity as provided by the American Epilepsy Society's annual meeting.

Chapter 3: Shaking Up the Legal Status of CBD Oil in the Cannabis Industry

The controversy continues over the legal status of the Cannabidiol (CBD) oil, but it is at this time legal in sixteen states. The benefits are too remarkable to be ignored. It is approved since research has indicated the patients won't be receiving the 'high' effects as with previous reports from marijuana usage.

This is a breakdown state-by-state:

Alabama: A million dollars has been allocated for the study of CDB oil at the University of Alabama. Governor Robert Bentley signed the Carly's Law on April 1, 2014, making it the second state to legalize the oil. The bill was so named for a three-year-old Carly Chandler who was sponsored by Senator Paul Sanford. It provided research for treatment for epilepsy, making it possible for the UAB to prescribe the oil to a list of approved patients.

Florida: The bill, HB 843, passed the House Judiciary Committee on April 22, 2014, which called for four organizations statewide to 'grow, test, and dispense' the oil. As the ninth state to legalize the oil; it would not be limited to seizure conditions; it could also be used for cancer, PTSD, Alzheimer's, and Parkinson's patients.

Georgia: The bill, HB885, is named for the four-year-old Haleigh Cox and is known as the Haleigh's Hope Act. On March 25, 2015—the House passed the bill to cover eight conditions including ALS, MS, sickle cell, mitochondria, cancer, and seizures. Georgia was the thirteenth state to legalize the CBD oil.

Iowa: It is legal to possess 32 ounces (a six-month supply). On April 9, 2014, the CBD oil bill passed calling for a study to be provided by the University of Iowa. The oil can be acquired in Colorado (presumed). This is the eighth state to legalize the oil.

Kentucky: SB124 placed Kentucky as the third state to legalize CBD oil on April 11, 2014. The oil is being researched at the University of Louisville and the University of Kentucky medical schools. It provides the CBD hemp oil to its patients enrolled in the trial program.

Mississippi: As the fifth state to legalize the oil on April 17, 2014; the bill allows the National Center for Natural Products Research located in Oxford to produce the medical oil.

Missouri: May 1, 2014, brought Missouri to the ranks as the eleventh state to legalize the oil which will direct the state's Department of Agriculture to provide a system under Health and Senior Services guidelines (non-profit). It is for patients who have suffered from seizures, and other regimens have not worked for them.

North Carolina: The state passed the bill on June 27, 2014 placing North Carolina tenth in the legalization line. Duke, Wake Forest, East Carolina, and UNC are providing studies to make the oil available for children who suffer from seizures. Neurologists will provide the medicine for the studies.

Oklahoma: As the fourteenth state legalizing the oil on April 30, 2015; it was decided to be used for children with 'debilitating' seizures.

South Carolina: The University of South Carolina is providing a clinical trial which began after the bill passed on May 28, 2014.

Tennessee: A research program has been directed to the Tennessee Tech University to study the efficacy of the oil used to prevent seizure activity. The school is also ordered to provide the oil to other schools of medicine. As the sixth state to legalize the oil; it is indicated the research must be completed by 2018.

Texas: The bill SB339 was signed into law on June 1, 2015, making the state of Texas the fifteenth state to make the oil legal. However, the bill differs from others because the oil must be consumed under specific guidelines.

Utah: The first state to legalize the oil was placed into effect on March 25, 2014. Low-THC industrial hemp can be grown by the Department of Agriculture for the purpose of the oil. The bill allows the residents of Utah to acquire the oil in Colorado and bring it home to Utah.

Virginia: The version of SB1235 placed Virginia as the twelfth state to legalize the CBD oil on February 26, 2015. It prevents prosecution for patients who are using the oil for seizure-related conditions.

Wisconsin: AB726 was in effect on April 16, 2014, making the state of Wisconsin the fourth legalized state for CBD oil. The details are ongoing.

Wyoming: The House Bill 32 became effective making Wyoming the sixteenth state to legalize the oil on June 30, 2015. The Department of Health can create a confidential database by creating hemp extraction registration cards. This will be effective after the physician determines the patient qualifies for the cannabidiol usage.

The status of Idaho and New York are still pending.

CBD Schedule 1 Drug

The controversial topic of cannabidiol oil continues as it is used by hundreds of thousands of patients within the United States for medical purposes. It is designated as a Schedule 1 drug according to the DEA.

The question rolls of how the CBD from hemp can fall within those guidelines? The Federal Register stated a new code number for 'marijuana extract' which pertains to any 'extract that contains one or more cannabinoids' that have been derived from any of the genus plant, cannabis. However, patients can avoid prosecution in the 28 states and DC.

These are the states where medical marijuana is legal:

- *Alaska*
- *Arizona*
- *Arkansas*
- *California*
- *Colorado*
- *Connecticut*
- *Delaware*
- *Florida*
- *Hawaii*
- *Illinois*
- *Maine*
- *Maryland*
- *Massachusetts*
- *Michigan*
- *Minnesota*
- *Montana*
- *Nevada*
- *New Hampshire*
- *New Jersey*
- *New Mexico*
- *New York*
- *North Dakota*
- *Ohio*
- *Oregon*
- *Pennsylvania*
- *Rhode Island*
- *Vermont*
- *Washington*
- *Washington, DC*

Where does the line get drawn?

It seems that it all depends on whether the oil has any traces of THC. Under that circumstance; most countries in the world would make hemp oil legal.

You can legally purchase CBD Oil derived from industrial hemp in the following states:

- Alaska
- Arizona
- Arkansas
- California
- Colorado
- Connecticut
- Delaware
- Florida
- Georgia
- Hawaii
- Idaho
- Illinois
- Indiana
- Iowa
- Kansas
- Kentucky
- Louisiana
- Maine
- Maryland
- Massachusetts
- Michigan Minnesota
- Mississippi
- Missouri
- Montana
- Nebraska
- Nevada
- New Hampshire
- New Jersey
- New Mexico
- New York
- North Carolina
- North Dakota
- Ohio
- Oklahoma
- Oregon
- Pennsylvania
- Rhode Island
- South Carolina
- South Dakota
- Tennessee
- Texas
- Utah
- Vermont
- Virginia
- Washington
- West Virginia
- Wisconsin
- Wyoming

The legal issues continue, making it a patchwork of what each state law indicates, which do not always conform to the federal standards.

Legalities in Germany

Several options are stated for legalities of cannabis usage as a medicine. It has been marketable since 2011. The cost of Sativex, a proprietary medicine, is approved for patients in Germany with Multiple Sclerosis with spasticity. The price can be covered by German health insurance companies. Also, a synthetic tetra-hydro-cannabinol (THC) is available through a private prescription.

However, at the person's own expense and a necessary permit, cannabis flowers are available from the pharmacy and are produced by a Dutch firm, Bedrocan. A certificate of exception must be sought from the Federal Institute for Drugs and Medical Devices.

UK Legalities

Areas of the United Kingdom - Wales, Northern Ireland, Scotland, England, and Great Britain grow industrial hemp with its 0.2% THC. It listed CBD as a medicine on November 2016 with regulatory control provided by The Medicines and Healthcare products Regulatory Agency (MHRA).

The issue is still debatable for cannabis as a Schedule 1 substance under the Misuse of Drugs Regulations of 2001. The ruling deals with substances which are perceived as not having any recognized medicinal values. This is an obvious contradiction to the MHRA ruling. Time will tell.

It is also illegal in the UK to give medical advice or medicinal claims regarding cannabidiol unless you have a license issued by MHRA.

UK residents of other European Union (EU) states who have signed up to travel with the prescribed psychotropic or narcotic substances, including cannabis into the UK, can travel from their own country according to Article 75 of the Schengen Agreement.

Legality of Sativex in the United Kingdom

GW Pharmaceuticals manufactures Sativex, a cannabis-based medicine. It is a palliative drug for cancer pain management as well as a spasticity reducer for those who suffer from Multiple Sclerosis.

As of 2006, the Home Office licensed the product so it can be legally dispensed in pharmacies and doctors can prescribe it to patients. As of April of 2013, Sativex was separated from cannabis; Schedule 4 (i) now applies.

Slovakia Legalities

The handling, import, and export from the Slovak Republic will require consent from the Ministry of Health, according to the guidelines set by the Slovak Parliament in 2011. The Psychotropic Substances Act ruled CBD into Group 2.

The ruling was essentially for the drug Sativex, which contains both CBD and THC. The Slovak Parliament claimed they were unaware that Sativex contained any CBD. Unfortunately, they still refused to remove the cannabinoid from Group 2.

New Zealand and Australia

It is legal, currently, to ingest hemp oil products according to the Food Standards Code of Australia/New Zealand (FSANZ) and the Therapeutic Goods Administration (TGA). In most Australian states except for NT, ACT, and SA allows hemp seed production if under license. On the other hand, hemp oil ingestion is outlawed according to FSANZ, but ingestion in NZ is permitted under specific circumstances.

Arrested or Not?

Many elements are involved as to whether you will be arrested or prosecuted for possession of the wonderful drug, CBD oil. Some of those issues are noted here:

1) If crossing an International border, whether you have nothing to declare or do not declare the oil or similar product you are carrying; you could be in trouble. For example, in Australia, if a hemp product has been declared, you probably won't be prosecuted, but the product will most likely be confiscated.
2) It may depend on whether you have a legal medical marijuana card or have a doctor's prescription in your possession.
3) It needs to be questioned whether you are allowed to carry/in your possession an amount of legal non-psychoactive or allowed legal medical cannabis.
4) It will be governed by on whether possession is decriminalized.
5) It will be decided how much THC is allowed; 0%, 0.2% or 0.3%.
6) It can depend on the source of the plant whether Industrial hemp or CBD oil products.
7) A huge factor will depend on the technical details of the local cannabis laws.

Chapter 4: CBD Oil Dosages

As with any medication, you need to know what amounts can be taken safely. Everyone is different, and the information provided is merely a guideline or a starting point for your new experience. As with any other medication; it is best to start with small doses and increase as needed.

Even with the beginnings of the legalization of the medical marijuana, physicians are also reluctant to prescribe the 'new' drug to patients. Medical scientists are currently developing schedules for the medical marijuana, and their extracts which include the CBD oil.

Its forms and concentrations vary and can be found as a thick paste, oil sold in capsule form, liquid hemp oil, and salves for topical use as well as tincture sprays or drops. A popular tool is the CBD vapor similar to the 3-cigarettes.

According to the Mayo Clinic, the Cannabinoid dosage will depend greatly on the type of disease. These are some of the guidelines on the topic:

Ailment	Amount of Dose
Chronic Pain	CBD is taken by mouth: 2.5 to 20 mg. each day for approximately 25 days.
Glaucoma Treatment	CBD taken under the tongue: 29 to 40 mg. (Over 40 mg. may cause pressure increases)
Increase the Appetite of AIDS and Cancer Patients	Taken by mouth: 2.5 mg THC (With or without 1 mg of CBD for 6 weeks)
Epilepsy	200 to 300 mg. CBD by mouth for

	4 ½ months
Movement Issues in association with Huntington's Disease	Taken by Mouth: 10 mg per kilogram of CBD each day for 6 weeks
Schizophrenia Treatment	Taken by Mouth: 40 to 1,280 mg CBD up to 4 weeks
Treatment of Multiple Sclerosis Symptoms Treatment	Plant extracts containing 2.5 to 120 mg of CBD-THC combination by mouth 2 to 15 weeks. A mouth spray may contain doses including CBD of 2.5 to 120 mg and 2.7 milligrams of THC for up to 8 weeks. *Note*: Most patients use a maximum of 48 sprays in a 24-hour period or 8 sprays within 3 hours.
Treatment of Sleep Disorders	40 to 160 mg. CBD by mouth

The most common application is an oral dosage with the use of drops/tincture or in a concentrated paste form. You need to hold the oil under your tongue so it can be absorbed in your mouth before you swallow. This is an essential step since part of the CBD is broken down by your digestive system.

You can also take the oil in the form of a chocolate bar, mouth strips, or the easiest form of a capsule. Other individuals enjoy using the inhalers or vaporizers. You can also find creams, balms, and lotions. The list is extensive of the many ways to take in the CBD oil; it will depend on what way you want to achieve the ultimate goal.

Varied Opinions

If you ask twenty different cannabis experts what the correct dosage for the oil should be; you will probably get twenty different answers. After all, with all of the government regulations and the lack of research in humans. Cannabis is by virtue a natural plant and contains many terpenoids, flavonoids, cannabinoids, as well as many other compounds.

CBD like cannabinoids are fat-soluble compounds which is how they taper off slowly and have prolonged effects. That is how so many drug screens are failed with the ingestion of cannabis. It is also believed men are less sensitive to the cannabinoids because women have a greater proportion of body fat in comparison.

Even in extreme doses of 700 mg to 1,500 mg daily, CBD shouldn't be toxic. There is, currently, no known fatal overdoses involving any cannabis products.

Chapter 5: What Makes CBD Different Today

In today's global society with the Internet as a resource; there are countless supplements offered as a calming and soothing medication. However, CBS is in a class alone with the possibility of more applications of the benefits of the oil usage in the near future.

Many individuals have found the CBD products as a welcomed relief to his/her daily life. Each person is different, meaning your needs may be different compared to a friend who is currently using one of the CBC products.

Rick Simpson Oil versus CBD Oil

Rick Simpson Oil became popular after the successful documentary, *"Run from the Cure"* while the anti-tumor effects provided by cannabis wasn't mainstream knowledge until 'the cat was out of the bag.' It has been deemed by Rick Simpson and many others as a cancer cure. Because of legalities of marijuana and cannabis, few clinical studies have been provided at this time. Looking toward the future; things are rapidly changing.

The Rick Simpson Hemp Oil Story

As a Canadian engineer who suffered from a constant ringing in his ears from a traumatic injury, discovered none of the doctors could discover a prescription that worked for the problem. After viewing an episode in the show *"The Nature of Things,"* Rick discovered a plan of extracting the oil from the plant to treat his ailment. It worked, and he was able to receive lowered blood pressure, and the pain was under control.

As time progressed, he developed some spots which were discovered to be skin cancer. As he recouped from the surgeries, he remembered a report from 1974 about THC and the treatment of cancer cells with the use of mice. As an afterthought, he applied the oil to the spots and discovered a few weeks later; the skin was healed.

He began handing out his oil to cancer victims at no cost to them, resulting in many being cured. However, the medical professionals were not as content with the 'cure.' He then decided on his documentary of *"Run From the Cure."*

Both oils are made from the cannabis/respectively hemp plant belonging to the same plant genus. However, through breeding and geographical factors, the plant has veered off into different strains and species. This produces a different type of harvest.

Hemp produces small flowers with low cannabinoid content, but the hemp provides fiber.

Cannabis, on the flipside, is a medical and recreational plant producing potent and large cannabinoid flowers with small amounts of fiber.

Whereas, the Rick Simpson oil is made primarily from the Cannabis Indica strains which are more effective for physical issues and ailments. Once again, on the other side of the coin, the Sativa strains are often time made into the Rick Simpson oil that is useful for mental illnesses.

This is a comparison of the two strains:

Top 5 Indica Strains

The Indica strain stimulates your appetite, reduces inflammation, and helps relieve seizures and spams. It is also an excellent sleep aid, stress and anxiety reducer, to relieve aches and pains. It will make you feel 'laid back' and relaxed.

- *Northern Lights* is a popular choice with its citrus sweet and earthy tone. It is considered 90% to 95% Indica. It is known for relieving the pain from anxiety, stress, insomnia, and other pain issues.

- *Critical Kush* has a pine 'skunky' taste that will produce a heavy-weight body stone. It generally packs 25% THC content and 2.1% of the CBD content.
- *Hindu Kush* originated in Pakistan and India and is considered the 'old-school' strain. It is known for lifting your mood as a 100% pure Indica strain. It is not as powerful as the Critical Kush.
- *Kosher Kush* contains an 80% Indica content which won the High Times Medical Cannabis Cup in 2012. You will receive a relaxing and deep body stone in the sense of euphoria and happiness.
- *L. A. Confidential* is an award winner of about 95% pure Indica. It bears a piney tone that will induce a peaceful mood and dispel your anxieties.

Top 5 Sativa Strains

Some of the general traits of the Sativa strand include the relief of depression, stimulation of the appetite, relief of nausea, migraines or headaches. You will also have a more uplifting and energizing feeling and feel like you are in a state of well-being. These are the ones which support this:

- JH (named after the "Emperor of Hemp") with a varied THC level of 20% to 24%.
- *Sour Diesel #2* carries a sour pack of 16% THC levels.
- *Kali Mist* is bred by the Dutch which is well liked by women with its pure 90% sativa strain. It packs in a punch of 22% THC.
- *Amnesia Haze* is well known by its name winning the High Times Cannabis Cup in 2004. The haze revels in lemony and sweet earthy undertones packing a 22% THC factor.
- *Train-wreck* is almost at 90% sativa genetic to create a high-intensity buzz that will slowly fade.

These plants may not have the same names in all cases, but you get the idea of how different the products are in comparison. Since they are from different strains (cannabis and hemp); they will naturally contain varied amounts of the cannabinoids.

The full spectrum plant extracted from cannabis for the Rick Simpson oil contains 'high' THC levels and other cannabinoids, (yes the word 'high' again). The THC ranges are easily fifty to sixty percent depending on the strain used. The CBD would probably range only ten to fifteen percent. Concentrated amounts of CBG and CBN may also be present.

On the other side of the spectrum, the CBD oil contains the high levels of CBD but only trace amounts of similar cannabinoids including CBN or THC.

Unfortunately, consuming large amounts of the CBD oil (olive oil based) is a digestive and expensive challenge. If the oil is affordable, it would still not meet the wider range of cannabinoids which are part of the spectrum of extracts provided in the Rick Simpson oil.

The Rick Simpson hemp oil is still unavailable in most localities because it contains THC. However, it does leave cannabidiol as an alternative.

Dravet Syndrome and Charlotte's Web

The debilitating disease of children's epilepsy prompted parents to use medical marijuana to remedy the seizure activity. Researchers at the University of Colorado have provided studies of genes with the type which causes Dravet Syndrome. The gene used was from Charlotte's Web, a strain of medical marijuana. The study is meant to explain why some patients received positive outcomes, whereas others did not.

The *Realm of Caring*, a non-profit organization, had five brothers who grew a plant that is remarkable since it was high in CBD without the psychoactive effects of THC (low quantities). The oil was named after the first young girl, Charlotte Figi, who received treatment using the new strain back in 2013.

While circumstantial evidence proposes Charlotte's Web can be exceedingly effective in treating conditions such as this, scientific investigation of the product has been stalled by the Federal drug laws that have strictly limited marijuana research.

After she began taking the miracle from the cannabis plant, her seizures dramatically declined. Many families continue to move to Colorado to access Charlotte's Web for their children since many areas will not allow transporting the oil across state lines, even to others where they use marijuana for medical purposes.

Chapter 6: What is On Today's Market?

One of the most important factors you need to consider before you decide to purchase CBD oil is to know how much CBD is packaged in each product, in other words, how much volume. You need to be sure it relates specifically to CBD and not just hemp oil.

The concentration refers to the total abundance of CBD when compared to the total volume of the product. New users generally take one to two mgs at first depending on your body weight, metabolism, and the desired effects. You can always add more once your body gets adjusted to this intake amount.

It might take some time to adjust, so taking it daily as a multivitamin supplement would provide the maximum efficiency. Give it about a week before you attempt to make the adjustments. If you use other products, you need to consider different products provide unique benefits and each has limitations.

This is just a list to let you know which oil products are available on the worldwide web:

CBD Oil: This is the strongest product you can purchase and is highly concentrated in the purest form. It comes in a variety of strengths which can suit all types of users. The flavor is left out because of the 'purity factor.' It can also be mixed with other foods, especially ice cream. Just don't panic if you are a beginner; the hemp oil usually comes in a syringe form.

CBD Gum: This is a convenient and inconspicuous method but does have a minty or strong hemp taste. You can remove any embarrassment of using a vaporizer or taking a pill. You have no worry because they contain natural flavors along with very few additional sweeteners.

CBD Vaporizers: A small e-pen can be used with a USB chargeable unit. The unit heats up and the CBD turns the liquid to an inhaled vapor. You will only need to purchase the vaporizer once. The cartridges will include the oil and are refills for the vaporizer unit. This form is much easier and safer for your oral tract and lungs since they do not create smoke, only vapors.

Vaporizing does not burn the flower the way smoking does since smoking releases the toxins which are so much like cigarettes. One study indicated the marijuana levels of ammonia were twenty times higher than that found in tobacco smoke. However, researchers stated it could have been an effect from nitrogen-based fertilizer used when the cannabis was grown. Who knows?

Don't be offended if a friend or co-worker thinks you are smoking unless you want them to know your secret. It is nothing to be ashamed of if you vape in public (if it is legal). After all, the UFC fighter, Nate Diaz, admitted on television in 2016 that he 'vaped' to help with inflammation and to aid the healing process. He chose the discreet way to deliver the needed cannabinoids.

CBD Tinctures: These are the most versatile and popular form which can be absorbed under your tongue with a dropper. You can experience peppermint, vanilla, and cinnamon to name a few. You can add it in a drink which can offer some variety. If you don't care for the flavors, you can always choose some of the CBD topical choices.

CBD Capsules: High concentrations of CBD and lower hemp oil are available as a standard dissolvable capsule. The superb feature is that they are odorless and tasteless. You can also keep a better record of how much you have consumed in one day.

If you decide you need to tweak the serving size; it may be a bit more difficult. You could resolve the issue by using another product such as a concentrated CBD tincture along with the capsules once you understand the dosages.

CBD Topicals: You can put the balms, lotions, creams, and other topicals right where you need to pinpoint the inflammation and stiffness. The unfortunate part is they do work slowly and tend to be a bit pricier. This is because they don't contain all of the ingredients found in traditional CBD hemp oil products.

Availability and Prices

Sativex was the first prescription medicine derived from cannabis produced by GW Pharmaceuticals. The spray is approved in New Zealand, Canada, Spain and the UK to patients who have spasticity because of multiple sclerosis. In Canada, it is also approved for advanced cancer pain and neuropathic pain. However, at this time, it is not available in the United States.

The subject of price and amounts are finally at hand. You will soon discover from this company (remaining unnamed) has to offer for CBD Oil products. The oils offered are 100% natural based or pure CBD paste, and oils refined with natural vegetable oils such as hemp oil or extra-virgin olive oil. All oils are consumable in foods or directly under the tongue.

This list is provided by the most popular choices:

Organic CBD Oil in the 10 ml size provides 4% CBD.
Priced at €27.5 or about $30 in U. S. currency. The cannabis used is bred to contain higher levels of THC but has been diluted until legal restrictions are met.

This is purely one example to show the expense which can be involved with the oils.

Consider the size of the bottle as to how many drops it contains. As a rule of thumb, generally there are about 500 drops in a one-ounce bottle.

Why it is So Expensive

The reason the CDB oil is so expensive hinges on several facts. There are many phases, and a considerable amount of plant material is required to harvest the oil. First of all, it takes many months to grow and harvest a sizable amount of hemp to produce enough seeds and stalk to harvest a very small amount of hemp extract.

At that point, testing begins to ensure its purity and compound composition. The extract is then transported into various forms of products, such as Vaporizer Oil or CBD Oil Drops. It is then placed on the line and is sold to retailers.

Each of the entities along the path grasps a fair profit for their efforts. By the time you have four or five of these entities involved; the cost has increased, making it what you see in the pricing market in this day and time.

You can compare the prices by breaking down each of the products into a cost per milligram of CBD. By performing this task; you can begin to make a comparison of the prices of each of the products. You must also consider that various brands focus on various characteristics.

The Best Method to Consume the CBD Oil

There is really no set rule concerning whether you extract, vape, or use the oil drops. Most beginners start with the drops and discover what other choices to make if he/she likes the effect of the oil. The drops are also the easiest choice to determine the serving sizes, and can also be flavored. It will basically be trial and error until you decide what best suits your needs.

It is an important step to be sure the product/products have been tested for residual solvents, pesticides, or potency.

Why the CBD Oil Market is So Risky

You should now understand how purchasing CBD oil can create some very big issues. These are some of the main ones that have caused the industry to become so out of control.

It is easy for a company to use dishonest practices with labeling its products. It is fairly simple to create dosages in the bottles that do not reflect the true contents. Some companies have listed the mg dosage of the CBD hemp oil but not publish the strength of its active CBD.

As an example, Company B has only 25% CBD by weight; they label it has 100 mg. of CBD hemp oil. In actuality, the product has only 25% of the active CBD oil.

Quality Control and Regulations form a gray area around the CBD products. A former Dixie Botanicals employee, Tamar Wise, turned into a whistleblower when she blasted the company for its deceptive practices. The point is that with the vague regulations around CBD products, it makes sick customers at the risk of false advertisement scams.

The nature of the customer demographic: Sick patients, friends, and families:
The CBD companies could be targeting families who are just in a corner suffering and have no other alternatives. In desperation, they will purchase 'possibly' ineffective oil. This makes this type of family situation in the hands of greedy businesses.

Most of the oil, possibly all of it, still has to be imported from other countries. In this country, hemp farming is largely prohibited even though the federal government legalized hemp farming in 2014 using the Farm Bill Act. As a result, the limited supplies result in higher prices to compete against importing the oil from countries including Eastern Europe or China—mainly Romania.

The hemp cultivation environment is essential because its properties absorb contaminants from the soil where it is growing. If you do not have clean soil, it could contain mercury or lead. Where does it stop?

Seven Top CBD Brands Online

These products have not been approved by the FDA. Also known as industrial hemp extract, CBD has been studied and is still in its infancy, but these are some of the top companies you can trust:

Populum Premium Hemp Oil only uses hemp that has been grown in Colorado in the United States with a unique orange flavor. The extraction purity was higher compared to competitor products at 80% concentration. The company was established in 2016 and has third party lab results. It is also made with 100% natural ingredients and is available in tinctures.

Green Lotus Rich Hemp Oil also uses hemp grown in the United States in Colorado and offers multiple flavors including peppermint, lemon, and orange. This is the first commercial company to conduct CBD and hemp research with a top-tier university. You can purchase tinctures or capsules. This product also has third party lab results. Research is conducted with the Texas A & M University.

Hemp Meds offers non-genetically modified ingredients in the form of concentrate, tinctures, capsules, or topicals. There are never any herbicides, chemical fertilizers, or pesticides used. The company has been operational since 2012, and the hemp is imported from Europe with no special flavors listed.

Delta Botanicals uses hemp grown in the United States (Colorado) and sells the product in the form of vape and tinctures. It is available in unflavored, vanilla cream, peppermint, pineapple, mango, and citrus. Third party lab results are available.

C W Hemp was established in 2014 and use hemp grown in domestic Colorado, USA. Tinctures are offered in olive oil and mint chocolate flavors and also have third party lab results. The company conducts research with *Realm of Caring*.

Bluebird Botanicals was established in 2012 with its hemp imported from Europe. You can purchase it in the form of vape, topicals, or tinctures with no specific flavors offered with 3rd party lab results.

Plus CBD Oil ranges from concentrate, to capsules, topicals, and sprays. The company was established in 2012 and offer peppermint, and vanilla flavors for the sprays. Third party lab results are available with the hemp imported from Europe.

Latest News on the Miracle Drug

With the passage of the 2014 Farm Bill and the legalization of recreational and medical marijuana in Colorado, studies have already begun.

A study in 2015 revealed young adults with epilepsy also received improvements with the use of the oil. A study in 2016, uncovered the fact that hemp oil increased motor skills, communication, language use, and alertness in 66 epileptic children

Eighteen children with epilepsy were included in a 2016 study which had their seizure activity cut in half with doses of up to 50 mg of the CBD oil.

Forty-two patients with acute schizophrenia discovered the oil was as effective as the standard anti-psychotic amisulpride versus the 800 mg dosage of oil. There were fewer side effects which make this a better treatment option.

In a 2013 study, forty-eight volunteers discovered .32 mg of CBD oil relieved anxiety and stress in many situations. It also reduced the traumatic experiences and bad memories of post-traumatic stress disorder.

CBD Oil for Animals

You need to consider the same CBD oil that treats human ailments can also improve the quality of life of fish, mollusks, and mammals which have an endocannabinoid system. It is simply the system of the CB1 and CB2 receptors using the neurotransmitter 'Anandamine' which in essence means bliss.

Worldwide, but especially in Canada and the United States, extensive research is being conducted for the effectiveness of the oil in horses, dogs, and cats. Since it works for humans; it is always nice to know your pets can receive the same benefits if needed.

Palliative Care

It is always good to know your beloved pet can receive some oil so the final phase of its life can benefit with comforting care and some relief of the pain. It will help give the pets overall life and body some balance to carry through with the final steps.

Dosage and Concentrations

Don't worry about any side effects since it will not have any THC. Doses are different and in line with the animal's weight factor. If it is a choice of a final dose; it will be adjusted individually with the pet's medical provider.

For a cat or a dog, most doses include one drop once or twice as a food supplement. It may take a week with daily intakes before you notice any changes. After that time, if there has not been an increase, add another drop. You can purchase it in different strengths, meaning you won't need to purchase concentrated oil.

Put it in the pet food or in a treat form. It will be consumed through the gastrointestinal tract as well as the oral mucosa (a mucous membrane).

Benefits for the Animal

- Helps support the immune system
- Improves the neurological function
- Can reduce any chronic pain symptoms
- Comforting for final life stages
- Supports gastrointestinal tract
- Improves mobility issues
- Helps the pet relax and be calmer

Just for Fun!

Make yourself some Canna-butter. It is not hard to make since you have the oil. You can make it using a 'per serving' formula. For example:

2 grams 25% oil (500 mg of CBD) makes 8 tablespoons

The boiling point of CBD is between 320°F and 356°F. Use lower cooking temperatures since some of the CBD might evaporate. Stay between these ranges for the best results.

Be sure to store the finished product in a cool, dark space since cannabinoids are light and heat sensitive.

Infuse the Fat

Try this next time you want something to feel better and don't want to use other methods.

1) You begin by heating the starting material (either coconut or olive oil).
2) Add the CBD oil and stir until well blended.
3) Store in a sterilized, clean container in a cool dark place.

4) Use as any other recipe; just remember to count the per-serving quantities.

You need to realize cannabis oils will work well with savory or sweet recipes.
The recipe needs to contain an oil-based ingredient or fat that can infuse with the concentrate. The fats include nut or vegetable oils, shortening, lard, ghee, or butter. You can also use some cognac, rum or vodka (just a splash) if you are up to it. Beer and wine do not work as well as a carrier for the oil.

Be sure the concentrate has been lab tested and approved. You need to have all of the precautions covered since it is a pricey choice. But, you are worth it!

Make some Cannabis CBD Salve

You can use the carrier oil of your choice but many prefer to use a blend of olive oils, sweet almond, and coconut. The recipe will yield about ten ounces of salve. It would be beneficial to place them into two-ounce tins for safe storage. This is the process:

Ingredients

1 ounce beeswax
1 cup cannabis CBD infused oil
1 ounce refined Shea butter

Instructions
1) Use a double boiler or make one using a smaller pot over top of a larger one with a few inches of boiling water.
2) You can substitute the smaller pan for a glass Pyrex cup if needed.
3) Pour the oil into the smaller pot/cup and bring the water to a simmer.
4) Stirring often, pour in the beeswax using a skewer as a stir stick.

5) Once the wax is dissolved; blend in the Shea butter—stirring until dissolved.
6) Pour the salve into the waiting containers. It may take several hours to solidify.

What a great and thoughtful gift for anyone who might appreciate the aroma of fresh cannabis.

You can use the salve for skin issues, inflammation, and localized pain. The industry is finally recognizing the benefits of CBD oil, but the legislation seems to be putting breaks on the plans. However, if you can locate the products, it will be worth it!

Note: Unrefined Shea butter has a distinct aroma, but it can also be used with this recipe.

Conclusion

Thank for making it through to the end of the *CBD Hemp Oil: The Essential Guide to Cannabidiol;* let's hope it was informative and able to provide you with all of the information to satisfy your curiosity.

CBD has become the most highly sought after compound agent in the past few years which also received a great deal of publicity after the special "Weed" aired on CNN. Since they have been found in medical marijuana dispensaries, doctors' offices and similar locations with no medical card required.

Even though the endocannabinoid system of the human body is still not entirely understood, many researchers have concluded the brain receptors as well as the central nervous system are very well-equipped to absorb the cannabidiol quickly. This is good news since some of the immediate effects are experienced by the patients within just a few minutes of the first dosage.

Experiment and have some fun, while removing the pain and putting away some of the other issues that plague your lifestyle.

Finally, if you found this book useful in any way, a review on Amazon is always appreciated!

61850790R00031

Made in the USA
Lexington, KY
22 March 2017